NERVOUS BREAKDOWN

Signs, Symptoms, and Treatment

John Smith

CONTENTS

INTRODUCTION

Nervous breakdown can be referred to as serious strike of psychological sickness. There are *numerous* reasons for nervous breakdown. These include stress, conflicting grief, unemployment, career burnout, death, breakup, being fooled by a beloved person, etc.

The psychological illness involves anxiety, severe stress, dissociation, psychosis, post-traumatic stress disorder, and depression symptoms from several factors in life.

Nervous breakdown is mainly used to identify those who are going through psychological sickness such as anxiety or depression. In the past, this condition was known as neuralgic disease, melancholia, neurasthenia, vapors, and prostration.

At first, all the medical experts and doctors thought of nervous breakdown as a problem of the nervous system. Afterwards, they noticed that the problem is a result of an ailment in the thoughts of the individual.

The categories nowadays consist of several medical diagnoses, which have been present in terms of manic break, panic attack, psychotic break schizophrenic episode, and post-traumatic stress disorder.

A patient is explained to have a psychological problem if he or she senses something that does not really happen in reality, has hallucinations, or hears voices. The signs of nervous breakdown are *different* from one person to another. The sufferer may also hear somebody say something, even if there is nobody existing in reality.

They have a tendency to be obsessive with doing something bad for them or anybody close by. Additionally, they begin to sense that they are offended or persecuted by other people while that does not really occur. These patients begin to have feelings of serious obligation or extreme elaborateness or unrealistic strong jealousy.

The other signs include *odd* dialog patterns which are not understandable since it is funnily structured and presented. The sufferers exhibit unusual manners that turn into being peculiar such as unusual body motions or disrobing actions in public.

Acceptable types of therapeutic interventions and psychotropic treatment have been implemented for the cure of breakdowns. Typically, the sufferers are reconditioned to previous performance or occasionally more desirable than before. This *depends* on the type of breakdown.

In certain cases of psychological illness, balanced body function can never be entirely reconditioned. Most of breakdowns observed in the last couple of years have been remedied by *suitable* treatment method that results in a fast restoration and protection against upcoming problems.

In this GUIDE, you will discover effective ways to survive your nervous breakdown and live a *stress-free* life.

Let us get started.

CHAPTER 1
WHAT IS A NERVOUS BREAKDOWN?

Nervous breakdown (or mental breakdown) is when the tension from stress gets so high that the mind and identity of a person break under the pressure.

How can stress, a thing which is not physical, break a person? Stress is a result of *inner* conflict: we feel like we have to do things we do not want to, and be someone we do not want to be. We try to delude ourselves and endure (this manifests as stress), but if we find no way to resolve this inner conflict, some part of us has to give up and break down.

When a person has a collapse, either emotionally or psychologically, it is often because of a nervous breakdown. A nervous breakdown is not a specific problem but a general term that covers a whole variety of mental illnesses.

People are typically diagnosed with it when they find themselves not able to exist in social roles that they once participated in. It is often accompanied by feelings of inadequacy, depression and losing touch with what is real or not real. Many times it shows up after a person has been in a long battle with stress and did not deal with it when it should have been dealt with early.

This type of problem can make it difficult to deal with many social and work functions of your life and can occur without notice. Not only does a nervous breakdown attack your head, but it can exhaust you physically and emotionally, as well. It can leave you feeling exhausted, weak, confused, disoriented, worthless and even cause you to cry without notice.

Your self-esteem can take a hard hit while your confidence slides to an all-time low. Weight loss or weight gain is often another side effect of this type of condition. Catatonic posturing is a severe side effect that needs to be looked into by a doctor. It causes a person to be unable to move and obviously can be very dangerous in a variety of situations.

What breaks during a nervous breakdown is the *identity* of a person. It is the way we see ourselves and which determines how we interact with the world around us. The way we think, the way we feel, our behavior, our habits, etc. All together form how we see ourselves, and when this perceived identity is torn apart all left are pieces.

A nervous breakdown forces us to look deeply within and create a better *"self."* It is possible to stay in the limbo of being broken down, but not for long. Even if you do not put the pieces together consciously, your subconscious will start doing the job for you.

The ignorant world does not understand how fragile the human conscience is and how *dangerous* the wild side of the human conscience is. The anti-conscience generates mental illnesses within our conscience.

A nervous breakdown is characterized by extreme stress. The individual feels that he or she cannot go on. The anxiety and the pressure of unbearable feelings transform his life into a nightmare. The absurdity that suddenly controls his mind is a force that surpasses his capacity to function normally.

Those who never had severe psychological problems cannot understand what happens with those who are suddenly obliged to deal with the unbearable symptoms of craziness, which are caused by the invasion of the anti-conscience into their human conscience.

Whenever an individual has traumatic experiences in life, his conscience will be unavoidably invaded by his primitive anti-conscience. This means that his human conscience starts listening to the absurd thoughts of his absurd and evil anti-conscience, while he believes that these thoughts belong to his human conscience.

This means that those who have traumatic experiences in life will unavoidably become mentally ill. They must follow the *right* psychological treatment; the natural treatment of the divine unconscious mind that produces our dreams with the intention to save our sanity and help us evolve.

People who believe that human beings are balanced and civilized rational animals are very far from the truth. Our capacity to think does not help us find peace and happiness because our thoughts are absurd. They are based on selfishness and evilness, even if we try to justify these thoughts with various excuses. We are constantly influenced by the absurd suggestions of our anti-conscience.

A nervous breakdown is caused by the pressure of the anti-conscience of an individual into his human conscience. The anti-conscience causes anxiety, panic attacks, dizziness, paranoia, and numerous abnormalities to the individual, who loses a big portion of his conscience. This pressure can be combated through dream therapy.

CHAPTER 2
THE UNDERLYING
CAUSES OF NERVOUS
BREAKDOWN

Life can offer us many challenges having to do with loss. When we are faced with relationship loss, financial loss, loss of health, loss of limb, loss of regard, or loss of love, we can feel overwhelmingly anxious, depressed and stressed.

When the anxiety, depression and stress get too big, we may have a nervous breakdown that we become incapable of functioning in our everyday life and incapable of coping with our daily challenges.

What causes one person to have a nervous breakdown while another, with equally difficult or even more difficult challenges, is able to stay functioning and even optimistic?

Imagine a seven-year old child trying to cope with a big loss in his or her life, like the loss of a parent. What enables the seven-year old to handle this loss? A seven-year old can handle the loss only when there is a loving adult helping him or her with the loss.

When there is no loving adult helping with the loss, the child may handle the loss by shutting down. The shutting down may lead to a loss of functioning, such as doing poorly in school.

However, when the child does not feel alone with the loss when there is love sustaining the child from an adult source, this child will be able to cope with the feelings of loss. The same is true for us as adults. We all have a very hard time with loss when we feel alone with it, but we can manage it when we are not alone.

However, we cannot always rely on others to be here for us in times of loss, stress and overwhelm. Those people who have family and friends always turn to for emotional and financial support during times of loss are fortunate indeed. But there are many people who are not so fortunate.

Without others to turn to, we need to be able to turn to a reliable inner source of love to make it through and not feel alone. This reliable source needs to be our inner spiritually connected loving adult self. Those people who are able to manage loss without losing functioning are those people who do not feel alone inside because they have developed a strong loving adult self.

I define the loving adult as the part of us that is open to learning from and connected with a spiritual source of love, wisdom, and guidance. It is the part of us that takes loving action in our own behalf, nurtures us when we feel fear and grief, and operates the truth from spirit rather than from the lies of our wounded self, our ego.

Just as children can manage loss when there is a loving adult to help them, the child in us can manage loss when we have a strong, spiritually connected loving adult self to help us. As a loving adult we know we are never alone. We know we are always being loved, sustained and guided by a spiritual source.

It is often not enough to have a strong religious or spiritual connection. If you have not been using that connection to develop your loving adult self, then there is no part of you to bring love and comfort to yourself when you most need it, and no part of you can take loving action for yourself, especially when things are overwhelming.

People who have nervous breakdowns are people who are not operating from a loving adult in their everyday lives. They are able to function as long as things go well, but when things fall apart, as they often do in life, these people may also fall apart. Without a loving adult to bring the love and truth of spirit to them, they end up feeling too alone to manage loss.

There are more than five ways to incite a nervous breakdown. In fact, the number is infinite, and certainly not limited to those noted below. Regardless of the way we go about it, the common theme among them is the same.

Each carries an unremitting burden of stress and anxiety which will eventually (either individually or collectively) break down our coping skills, and very often our immune system. The so-called "dysfunctional" feelings and actions that result may include hostility, anger, depression, sadness, substance abuse and many others.

For the sake of examples, here are five ways we can all promote our own nervous breakdown.

#1: Submitting to constant worry

Wasting time trying to figure out answers to problems that have not yet occurred.

#2: Constantly relive your past

Allowing your past to minimize, or destroy, your future.

#3: Avoid making decisions

Decisions will eventually be made for us (and often forced on us) if we do not respond to our responsibilities. One of our greatest freedoms is making our *own* decisions. Seems a shame to voluntarily allow others to make decisions for us.

#4: Place unrealistic demands on yourself

Do not beat your head against the wall. The wall does not change, and all you get out of it is a headache. Make progressive steps to achieve your goals. There is only *one way* to eat an elephant. One bite at a time.

#5: Allow negative influence from people masquerading as friends

Being unwilling to manage the kinds of people you allow into your life, or being unwilling to discern who has your best interests at heart. Pain is inevitable in this life, but misery is optional.

Everyone has a different threshold for what they can manage emotionally, before their coping skills fail them. To re-orient ourselves from the throws of stress and anxiety, we often search for ways to remove the influences causing us to be pushed closer and closer to, or over, our threshold.

CHAPTER 3
SIGNS AND SYMPTOMS
OF A NERVOUS
BREAKDOWN

A nervous breakdown is a largely utilized name in today's society, applied to explain a psychological disorder that an individual encounters.

It is utilized for an amount of causes, for example: to hide a diagnosis; to stay clear of the stigma of a diagnosis; not understanding the reasons for certain loss of function (such as not seeing a physician, but having signs or symptoms); and not recognizing a diagnosis among others.

The signs of nervous breakdown can *vary* from person to person, but I try to dissect them in this chapter.

Fundamentally, the signs of nervous breakdown are when *variables* one usually cannot regulate compound into one *factor*, and the individual feels as though crushed by inner thoughts. These include fearfulness, sadness, anxiousness, which can occasionally lead to feelings of suicide, or romantic ideas of starting a new life.

A nervous breakdown can be very *easily* averted, with appropriate comprehension of what fear and panic are, and with proper direction of one's everyday living. As a past victim myself, I can state that remedy can simply be gotten before you reach the brink. It is very important for you to do so before more severe consequences arise.

The effects of panic, anxiety, and eventually nervous breakdown can be debilitating. Both to one physically and mentally. They can ruin someone's life, dominate their thoughs, their mental processes, and thoroughly inflect themselves on people's life. The anguish could be taken out on your loved ones, lashing out at them for things they are not responsible for.

A nervous breakdown occurs when someone reaches a point of complete exhaustion after a protracted spell of anxiety. The anxiety could be caused by any number of factors: an unhappy romantic relationship, a worsening financial period, worries at work about whether you may lose your job. Perhaps a combination of all these things.

Indeed, it is unlikely that a nervous breakdown would be brought on by just one factor. It is usually when worry is piled on to worry that you find yourself headed down this most unpleasant path. Eventually, you find that you cannot deal with life anymore. It is all too much and you just want to stay in bed and make the world go away, to borrow the words of the song.

Sometimes, it can be just one more adverse event that sends the person into a tailspin; the sudden death of a loved one, or the sudden and totally unexpected loss of a job. Now, I can imagine the face of the actor **Liam Neeson** at the beginning of the movie *"The Commuter* (2018)." Like most mental conditions, except for the panic attack, which suddenly comes and slaps you around the side of the head, so to speak, there are definite symptoms.

The person does not want to eat. Sex is the last thing on their mind. Like depression, they have no further interest in hobbies or life in general. They may feel guilty for feeling the way they do. Then they may feel pathetic and this makes them feel even worse. Even the smallest task is way beyond them.

Feelings of being alone even in the bosom of their family. And desperation. If someone has had the misfortune to experience a nervous breakdown, they may become impatient with themselves, lose their confidence and not surprisingly, be afraid that there may be a repeat performance.

Nervous breakdown is a mental illness triggered by depression or anxiety and is faced by people worldwide. It is also termed as a mental breakdown. There are many factors contributing to such a dilemma but social isolation is the major cause and is quite irreparable.

A person might feel one or more of the symptoms listed below simultaneously or in an exaggerated form depending from one infidel to the next, from one's mental stability and past history of mental disorders.

Symptoms of a Nervous Breakdown

#1: Physical

A brain that is experiencing excessive stress like, feeling of lethargy, constant pains and aches, is showing signs of a nervous breakdown. Skin feels scratchy and inflamed, lowered body resistance and repeated sensations of vomiting. Major gastric problems come about like stomach cramps, gastrointestinal ulcers, colitis and diarrhea over extended periods of time are indicative of a nervous breakdown.

#2: Hostile behavior

An individual exhibiting signs of a nervous breakdown displays antisocial behavior like gambling, vandalism, and alcoholism. Some might even use drugs as an escape to lessen the pressure, though not a rule.

#3: Amnesia

Cases of short term memory loss like forgetting appointments and schedules, showing signs of confusion on the past order of events that describes amnesia, if left untreated leads to frustration, an added pressure to the brain, which results to rage and powerful displays of outbursts.

#4: Delirium

People show signs of delusions and visualize hallucination by tasting, seeing, feeling, and hearing things that are not there. They may have extreme cases of nightmares and are obsessed with terrors.

Panic attacks, sleepwalking, and morbid thoughts like harming or destroying other people, even committing suicide. Being very vain to the point of adoring oneself also is a person suffering from a nervous breakdown.

A person suffering from a nervous breakdown has a *totally* different personality from what he used to be. This absolute disruption of personality from a fixed normal and functional routine switches to a chaotic and disruptive lifestyle.

They cry and feel sad the whole time. They have low energy levels that are why they feel desolate. They suffer from insomnia so they cannot think.

John Smith

CHAPTER 4
HOW TO DIFFERENTIATE CHRONIC FATIGUE SYNDROME AND A NERVOUS BREAKDOWN

Chronic fatigue syndrome and a nervous breakdown are often thought of as a condition that is one and the same. However, both these are entirely different from each other. Here we differentiate the two by looking into their definitions, signs and symptoms and other pertinent information.

Chronic fatigue syndrome is a disorder that affects many people, a condition wherein the fatigue does *not* have a known cause and it occurs for a long period of time, for *six months* or even longer.

This is more common in females, especially those who are at the young and middle adulthood. The exact cause for CFS is not known but studies have found that it is often associated with infections and chronic diseases.

Chronic fatigue syndrome symptoms include fatigue for six months or more, cognitive difficulties such as short-term memory problems and inability to concentrate, headaches, joint pain that is accompanied by redness and swelling.

There can also be tenderness at the lymph nodes, sore throat and muscle pains. Other chronic fatigue syndrome symptoms are feeling tired even after sleeping and being extremely tired that lasts for more than *a day* after you have been doing some physical activities.

Treatment for CFS will depend on the chronic fatigue syndrome symptoms being manifested. Medications will be prescribed if the muscle and joint pain are intolerable, also for sleep disturbances and psychological problems.

Diet and nutrition can play a significant role in the improvement of CFS, and it is recommended that you should have an increase in the intake of *vitamin B6, B12* and *vitamin D*. Stress reduction therapies are also recommended as well as avoiding strenuous activities. Other treatment methods are cognitive behavioral therapy, graded exercise therapy and pacing.

Meanwhile, a nervous breakdown is used to describe a mental disorder experienced by a person wherein anxiety or depression is usually present. This disorder has various causes such as stress, problems with relationships, work, and school or with finances. It can also happen in those who have health problems such as chronic diseases like cancer.

A nervous breakdown can cause significant changes in a person's life such as decrease in concentration, sudden mood changes, loss of appetite and sleep disturbances. Other nervous breakdown symptoms are dizziness, insomnia, palpitations, having frequent nightmares and some may even have amnesia.

For a nervous breakdown to be treated, you must *first* acknowledge that you have a problem. Once you do that, you will be able to seek help and talk about the certain cause of your problem. You and your health practitioner will be able to formulate a treatment plan based on the causes of your nervous breakdown.

Aside from facing the problem, you will also need to do other therapies to treat a nervous breakdown and to prevent further episodes. Exercise, having a healthy diet, getting adequate rest, meditation, aromatherapy and avoiding smoking, alcohol and drugs are also helpful in treating a nervous breakdown.

Knowing the difference between a nervous breakdown and chronic fatigue syndrome will help you in identifying the *proper* treatment methods needed for your condition. This way, you will be able to have a *full* recovery without any complications.

John Smith

CHAPTER 5
HOW TO MANAGE ANXIETY AND A NERVOUS BREAKDOWN

What is the relationship between anxiety and a nervous breakdown? Phobias, panic, and obsessive-compulsive disorder are a few of the conditions that fall under the category of anxiety. The terms of anxiety disorder and situational depression have taken the place of the term nervous breakdown in the medical community.

Although occurrences in your life can be responsible for anxiety disorders; there are also genetic, biological, or neurological explanations for them as well. When an event in your life causes a specific reaction, or when mental illness comes on quite unexpectedly, these instances are typical of situational depression.

Trying to battle against situational depression may be making it more difficult for you to deal with a nervous breakdown or avoid having one in the first place.

You may need to identify the trouble spots in your life which are causing you to feel anxious and tense, especially if you are beginning to feel overwhelmed. Most individuals will tend to try to regain control when they notice that they are losing it.

You will need to make a concerted effort to find peace and serenity if you wish to get yourself back in control again after a nervous breakdown has occurred. When you continue to try to cope after you have already reached your physical or mental limit, you are allowing your anxiety to remain in control.

You can counteract the factors that caused your body and mind to react by having a nervous breakdown if you are prepared to let yourself have the feelings that you need to have in reaction to the event.

Seeking professional help carries with it the connotation that the nervous breakdown and anxiety have won the war. But, in reality, reaching out for help indicates that you are trying to help yourself to recover from your problems.

It is not necessary to continue to undergo therapy or get professional assistance forever. You will find that you do not need any further professional help when you are *aware* of what is responsible for your distress and pain, and you have the skills necessary to avoid similar situations in the future.

There is certainly a benefit to be gained by consulting a professional when you are first faced with anxiety and nervous breakdown, so that you do not experience long term harm.

CHAPTER 6
HOW TO PREVENT A
NERVOUS BREAKDOWN

There is *no* way to avoid the pressures of life. Merely living puts us under the pressures of survival. Your body demands sustenance and your lungs demand air. From the *very* moment of birth, pressures begin to mount.

We have pressure from our parents to grow up right, we have pressure from teachers to learn, we have peer pressures, we eventually have the pressures of relationships, of society, and of the workforce.

Pressure comes from *all* aspects of life. There is very *little* we can do to avoid it. As a pastor and a Christian, we talk about giving problems and cares to God. But this *Biblical* approach is misunderstood in this context. Giving things to God only relieves stress. It does not relieve the pressure.

For example, I want my children to grow up and become all they can be. I do not want them to be menaces to society. I want them to be decent, honest, good, and have access to all the joys in life available to them under God.

This pressure is the same no matter if I give my children to God or not. The desire to have them grow up right will not change no matter how I deal with it.

To avoid a nervous breakdown in life, you not only need to understand the pressures in your life, but you must have reason to be under it. Call it a cause. A cause is something that is greater than you. It is something beyond you. It is something that is motivational and driving.

People have nervous breakdowns because they cannot *find* a reason to live under the pressures of life. These pressures cause them to snap. They may seem okay one day, and the very next they go ballistic. People endure great hardships when they have a reason to endure them. Take the reason away, and they fall apart under the pressure.

- *What is your purpose in life?*
- *Why are you married?*
- *Why do you have children?*
- *Why are you going to work?*
- *Why do you do what you do?*

The answers to these questions, good, bad, indifferent, or weak will tell you if you are a candidate for a nervous breakdown or not. If, for example, you have *no* cause and the *only* reasons you do anything are purely selfish, then you are a candidate for a nervous breakdown.

Dust happens. Your house cannot exist in a vacuum, and that is why it has to be cleaned regularly. No matter how careful you are, dust will enter. Same with the mind. You desire to keep it quite and serene, but life kicks up mental and emotional noise and dust that needs to be dealt with. So, how do you deal with it?

The key is do *not* let it accumulate. As a storm gathers, so does stress. It is only when disorder or disturbances accumulate that they become overwhelming and feel beyond your ability to handle. It is much easier to clean a dusty house than a dirty house. Resolve or relax any disturbance on the spot.

Do not carry it over to the next minute, the next hour and especially not the next day. Stress prevents you from living the next moment free and clear. You lose clarity and power which diminishes your immunity to handle the next stressful situation, creating a thicker and thicker barrier to relaxation and recovery.

If you do not eat or drink too much today, you will not have a hangover tomorrow. If you let go of anger, resentment, fear, jealousy, etc., today, there is no foundation for it to grow or fester. Stressful thoughts or feelings are diseases that grow like any bacteria grows.

Stop them on arrival or prevent them from arising in the first place through constant diligence. Diligence is the *cost* of freedom from the accumulation of stress. Begin and end your day in a relaxed and detached way. Let the little dings and pressures of the day flow away from you, like water off a duck's back.

You cannot let your house go but you can let the dust go. Likewise, you cannot let life go, but you can let unproductive or negative thoughts and feelings go. Clean one room *at a time*, one thought or feeling at a time, one moment at a time.

Enter the moment in a state of calm acceptance of everyone and everything without thinking anything of it. If you can change it, do so; if not, drop it. This is the definition of love, wisdom and meditation. Be a lover, not a loser. Do not let the world suck you in.

Keep a respectable distance from it. The external world also consists of your thoughts and feelings. Yes, they are external to you, external to the higher you. Keep them that way. It is for you to overlook them, and never let them overlook you.

You can also prevent having a nervous breakdown and feel that you cannot think anymore, you cannot trust your own judgment, and you do not know how to deal with the outside world before being in such situation.

If you are always stressed, anxious, afraid, and depressed, you must urgently follow a psychological treatment. I can translate your dreams for you and provide you with psychotherapy. After my initial help, you will overcome your problems. Then, you will learn the dream language and keep translating the meaning of your dreams yourself.

You will verify that you should never take medications to eliminate panic attacks and all the unbearable symptoms caused by mental disorders. You must follow dream therapy and understand what is causing these abnormalities so that you may definitively stop having panic attacks and other unbearable symptoms.

It is a big mistake to stop having panic attacks with medication. If you cannot solve the problems causing panic attacks, you will *someday* have a nervous breakdown and be unable to function normally for an extended period of time. You may need *one year* to recuperate your conscience again after having a mental breakdown.

Medication does not work when you come to the point of having a nervous breakdown. It helps you forget your pain only in the beginning when you start having panic attacks.

This is why you must take dream therapy very seriously and eliminate all psychological problems and unbearable symptoms torturing your mind before having a nervous breakdown.

John Smith

CHAPTER 7
IDEAS TO HELP YOU
RECOVER FROM A
NERVOUS BREAKDOWN

Like bad dreams, nervous breakdowns do not last forever. Sooner we hope, rather than later, you are going to start to feel better. Now, you never know. Some of those terrible problems you have been worried sick about may have simply vanished like the *mists* of morning. Believe me, this can happen.

As to those that have not, though, make a list of them in order of importance and start to deal with them one at a time. You are feeling up to it. Tackle one problem at a time and at your own pace. Remember, you have just been sent a very strong signal by way of a nervous breakdown, which your life up to that point was not quite as it should have been.

Therefore, spend part of your relaxation and recuperation in deciding how different your life is going to be for you now. What changes are you going to make?

You often hear people boasting about the number of hours they put in at work.

"Oh, I am never happy unless I am working 80-hour weeks" or "If I only work a sixty hour week, I think I have been on holiday." How many hours a week did you work and look where you have ended up.

There are always occasions when we have to work long hours for a day or two, but make it a day or two, not permanently. How has your family been throughout all this? Perhaps more time spent with them would be an excellent idea for the future.

Take up *hobbies* that you have not touched for years. Something that challenges your mind, but in an entirely different direction from your normal occupation.

Personally, I started to write. I have always loved reading spy novels and I thought I would try my hand at writing one. In the event, it was a shambles, but at least it focused my mind on something other than my occupation. Well, that is not quite true. I was forced to retire. I was past retirement age in any case, but I would have visions of working well into my eighties.

Then, with my new found freedom, I thought I was being clever by pulling the odd all-nighter. Trying to write until dawn. That did not last long. I have simply become too tired for that sort of game these days.

Just for now, though, bear in mind that because you pushed yourself too hard, you jumped the tracks for a while. Now you are back on them again, set yourself strict limits about the hours you work, and the amount you take on.

As I said at the beginning, you must control your life, not the other way around. Obviously, it depends whether you are employed or self-employed, but whether it is the former or the latter, you are still under a doctor's care, so ease yourself back into work gently. Do not go charging back in like a roaring lion.

Two or three days a week are quite sufficient to start with, then as you keep feeling better, extend them to a full working week. However, remember now. You have had your warning.

John Smith

CHAPTER 8
NATURAL WAYS TO TREAT
NERVOUS BREAKDOWN
SYMPTOMS

Today, stress, anxiety, and depression are all at record levels. Consider all the stress we are subjected to; all the worries we have. All the secret fears we keep repressing that "something bad" is going to happen any minute. All the ominous news reports we listen to. It is an enormous wonder that more of us are not keeling-over in the middle of breakfast or having nervous breakdowns.

Nervous breakdowns occur when you have been living on your nerves for so long that you have effectively blasted your nervous system to pieces. As someone who has had at least nine nervous breakdowns so far this year, I now consider myself something of an expert on how to deal with them.

Every single health issue we have has *three* aspects, namely the spiritual aspect, the emotional aspect, and the physical aspect.

Let us run nervous breakdowns through our three-part diagnostic system, to see how we can start to strengthen our nervous system and hopefully limit our nervous breakdowns to only one a year.

#1: Spiritual health actions

When we do not believe in God, do not see his hand in the world, or do not believe that he is looking out for us, cares for us, and has our best interests at heart, this puts enormous amounts of stress on our system.

Just think about all the horrible things that could happen to you today: you could catch Ebola; you could get fired; your house could burn down - all terrible, horrible things.

But when we work on believing in God a bit more, and trusting him to take care of us, our spiritual stress starts to reduce, and we feel fundamentally more relaxed.

#2: Emotional health actions

You can sum it up like this: turn off the news, and stay away from negative, pessimistic people who are always trying to persuade you the end is nigh. Life is actually pretty good. Take a few minutes every day to count the blessings in your life, and say thank you.

You should make a *gratitude list*. **Oprah Winfrey** swears by it. If you like to read more about it, please check another book of mine, named *"Anxiety and Panic attacks."*

#3: Physical health actions

Bladder is the energy meridian that governs the nervous system. Anything you do to strengthen the bladder meridian will pay big dividends. Things that have worked for me include:

- Using *lavender* essential oil, and other sedative oils, to physically relax and de-stress tense muscles

- Sticking *lentils* on the acupressure source point for the bladder meridian (*seeds* contain a lot of innate healing energy)
- Using *acupressure points* to strengthen the flow of energy through the bladder meridian
- Quitting my horrible, deadline-driven, soul-destroying job

Experiment and see what works for you, and in the meantime, let me reassure you that nervous breakdowns, or nervous exhaustion, or neurasthenia does not have to take you out of action for years: if you follow the three-pronged approach outlined above, you could bounce back from your nervous breakdown in a matter of *hours*, not months.

To be honest, there are no single cures for a nervous breakdown as it can be caused from a variety of sources, and every single person is *different* after all. So one thing you can do is to see if one of these techniques will work for you.

Try breathing slower, slowly than usually and clear your mind of stressful thoughts.

Try turn on some music, or at least find a quiet area to envision yourself in a peaceful situation.

Calming music can help, also avoid drinking any caffeine or sugars in the future, as these will heighten stress level.

There are also natural herbs out there such as *valerian*, the *passion flower*, and tons of others that will help you find a better sense of peace in your situation.

John Smith

CHAPTER 9
TREATMENTS OF
NERVOUS BREAKDOWN

The nervous breakdown is one of the most feared of all diseases. People suffering in this way are described in many ways. Sometimes as people who have lost their mind or gone insane.

Conventional medical practice is to treat people with therapy, sleeping pills, antidepressants, psychotropic medication or even a stay in a mental hospital. The full NHS treatment of a "breakdown" reinforces the patient with the idea that they are "ill."

Nervous breakdowns are *not* an illness, they are the minds natural attempt to sort out historical memories and rebalance itself. The main problem arises because the mind needs *time* to go through this evaluation and healing process. Our society does *not* allow time for this, so one or several "quick fixes" are used.

When people lose control of their minds, they become frightened and resort to short term measures. If they cannot resolve their problems themselves they may resort to drugs or alcohol to get through the day.

It is now assumed that these mental periods of insanity are not actually a nervous breakdown but a person's period of mental reassessment. Sometimes these mental reassessments are triggered by life events which may not even be traumatic in themselves.

Normal mental reassessments are continually going on in the subconscious mind as it approaches every new day. But occasionally the mind is faced with confusion and disorder as it attempts to evaluate an unexpected situation.

It will then dig deep into its historical experiences and memories searching for the solution. During this period of self-analysis, the patient may become irrational, unable to continue with their normal life or work pattern and communicate abnormal thoughts and ideas.

Our inability to isolate ourselves from others also becomes a problem here. A close personal relationship could intrude into the natural healing process as could normal family life.

Also our ongoing natural dependence on the logical assessments made by our conscious mind can turn our brains into a battlefield where the conscious and the subconscious mind are fighting each other for control.

Alternate therapists allude to the fact that reprogramming the subconscious mind can take *40 days*. This is not dissimilar to the period of meditation suggested by Yoga teachers for cleansing the mind or the period of isolation required by Buddhists, Jesus, and Reiki philosophers.

So trying to attain a "quick fix" is ultimately self-destructive because resorting to drugs or alcohol will actually extend this period indefinitely. Mental reassessments can be completed in anything from a few days to a month when the patient is given the necessary guidance.

This guidance will probably involve alternate therapies offering counselling, relaxation, massage, and meditation.

First things first, if you have any of the following nervous breakdown symptoms now, skip to the bottom of this chapter for immediate relief.

- Racing heart
- Excess sweating for no apparent reason
- Full-blown panic attack
- Extreme muscle tension
- Thoughts of self-harm

If you are currently in a relaxed state and merely want to know about the symptoms and treatments for panic, read on. It is important to note that the term "nervous breakdown" is not an official medical term. It is rather a broad social term that covers many mental illnesses. Probably, the most common medical disorder associated with a nervous breakdown is chronic panic disorder.

Panic attack symptoms revolve around an intense fear that consumes the entire body. The symptoms generally start with an increased heart rate and breathing level. The panic sufferer will notice this and will possibly form fears that they are having a heart attack. This generally scares the person even more, and a full-blown panic attack ensues.

Panic attacks can occur at any moment, and are not necessarily brought about by a particular event. The underlying causes of the disorder are difficult to evaluate but are generally sourced from an underlying fear or generalized anxiety.

Immediate relief for nervous breakdown symptoms

- Sit still and actively force yourself to breathe slowly
- Stop all thoughts
- Close your eyes and imagine yourself lying on a comfortable secluded beach on a beautiful sunny day
- Continue to think about only this, and make sure you slow down your breathing

There may have been times in your life when you felt like you were having a "nervous breakdown." But what is a nervous breakdown? A nervous breakdown is a very broad and general term for various psychological problems and disorders. It is an unscientific term that the medical profession does not use anymore.

If you have chronic anxiety or depression, cognitive-behavior therapy is an excellent treatment. CBT attempts to change distorted, negative thinking patterns, and unwanted behavior. It usually includes exposing individuals to feared situations. CBT is very effective and one of the best treatments for anxiety disorders and other unhealthy conditions.

If you have ever felt like you were having a "nervous breakdown," you could have been having a panic attack or very anxious.

Here are five steps that will help you to deal with panicky feelings or "waves of anxiety."

#1: Accept and allow anxiety

First off, acknowledge your anxious feelings. Then accept and allow your anxiety. Do not try to "fight" your anxious feelings and symptoms or pretend they are not there. Instead, accept and allow yourself to feel anxious. Tell yourself statements like "It is okay if I am anxious," "It is not a big deal to have anxiety" and "I am just anxious because..."

#2: Do deep breathing

Do not forget to breathe. Inhale through your nose to the count of four *slow* seconds. As you inhale, you should feel your belly expand like a balloon being filled with air. As you do this, try to keep your shoulders and chest movement at a *minimum*.

While your belly is still expanded, hold your breath for a couple seconds. Now you are ready to exhale. Open your mouth and exhale for five or six slow seconds. As you do this, your belly move inward. Do this type of breathing for a couple of minutes.

If you want to learn more about meditation, please check my book named *"Meditation for Beginners."*

#3: Pinpoint

If you can, try to pinpoint what triggered your anxious feelings and what it is bothering you. Are you anticipating something that is coming up? Have you taken on more than you can chew? Having an obsessive thought? Are you doing a lot of "what-if" thinking? Are you feeling guilty for something you should not? Are you being a *perfectionist*?

#4: Positive thoughts

Tell yourself positive things to help you get through this anxious episode. Most people have no idea how much their thoughts affect how they feel. You could tell yourself statements such as *"It is not a big deal that I am anxious. My anxiety will not harm me."*

Most people will not be able to tell *"I am anxious."* This anxiety will pass, it always does. Try to make your positive self-talk comforting and specific to the situation you are dealing with. Also, try to find a bit of humor in the situation. Learn to *not* take yourself so seriously.

#5: Do something

Distract yourself physically and mentally. Your body is ready to *"fight or take flight."* Do something with the adrenaline in your body. Do some type of physical activity for about fifteen minutes or longer.

CONCLUSION

◆ ◆ ◆

We live in a *stress-filled* society. Work, home, unemployment, marital issues, family, school, finances are just a few things than can raise our anxiety levels. On the other end of the spectrum, there is also severe depression, and for some people there is both. Sometimes it gets so overwhelming that it leads to an acute attack - commonly known as a nervous breakdown.

Feelings of extreme stress and anxiety do not go away. This may be accompanied by muscle pain or aches, a tired worn out feeling, stomach cramps and even ulcers. Secondly, the person may start displaying behavior out of character and antisocial, and they might also increase consumption of alcohol or narcotics.

Some people on the verge of a nervous breakdown could even start to show symptoms of delirium, such as hallucinations or seeing and hearing things that do not exist except in their minds.

Others might suffer from amnesia, although usually mild in nature. This includes short term memory loss and constantly forgetting things. This, of course, leads to more anxiety and stress.

In extreme cases symptoms could include an obsession with the occult, suffering from panic attacks and a deep feeling of depression along with thoughts of suicide. At this level, the sufferer can become a risk factor to not only themselves, but to society in general. There is no doubt that a complete nervous breakdown is imminent, and the patient needs immediate help.

Basically a nervous breakdown means that you are not able to function correctly in your day-to-day life after some kind of an event. Perhaps you feel like you have reached a limit to what you can do for yourself, and you see no way to get back to the way you used to be.

Whatever the case may be, there could be something like anxiety or depression can make you more nervous than most people. Generally, you need to get those things fixed if you want to get rid of the chance that you will have a nervous breakdown.

It is very important for you to remember that you should call a suicide hotline or tell someone if you feel like hurting yourself or other people. You can even take yourself to the hospital and let them know what is going on and they will be able to get you the help you need.

It can be expensive if you go to the hospital, but that is nothing compared to what could happen to you if you decide to take your own life or try to hurt another person due to your mental state.

You may want to start going to counseling and even maybe get on some medications. Generally, you have to see someone different to work on your medications, and then you can see someone that you can tell all of your problem.

Whatever the case may be, it is always a good idea to figure out what to look for when you are taking medications in terms of side effects.

Many people have a hard time dealing with these side effects, so they have to switch medications. Do not be afraid to bring up medication changes to a doctor because their job is to make sure you are on something that works for you.

Try to keep yourself away from stress for a while when you feel like you are at your breaking point. When you have a nervous breakdown, it is generally because you are too stressed out and have too much on your plate to do.

If you can, take a little while off of work and make sure that you have someone do your house chores for you if possible. Just try to take it easy because this kind of a breakdown is your body's response to a lot of stress.

Now it is probably easy for you to tell if you are having a nervous breakdown or if you know someone that has. This is not going to be easy to get through, but know that it will end and you will be able to get help if you need it.

After applying these treatments that mentioned above in this BOOK, if you do not see any improvement (a few hours to 40 days), it is time for you to seek help.

For those who have been seeing an increased level of stress and anxiety in themselves or others, should contact a professional for help and treatment. There are medications along with therapy that can do wonders and give those feeling like they are headed for a nervous breakdown finally feel some relief.

Printed in Great Britain
by Amazon

31232338R00030